Medical Marijuana Rules and Procedures

What U.S. states have legalized medical marijuana?

Alaska

Arizona

Arkansas

California

Colorado

Connecticut

Delaware

District of Columbia

Florida

Hawaii

Illinois

Louisiana

Maine

Maryland

Massachusetts

Michigan

Minnesota

Missouri

Montana

Nevada

New Hampshire

New Jersey

New Mexico

New York

North Dakota

Ohio

Oklahoma

Oregon

Pennsylvania

Rhode Island

Utah

Vermont

Washington

West Virginia

Medical marijuana is legal in 33 U.S. states and the District of Columbia by affirmation of a qualifying condition or prescription from a licensed physician.

Medical Marijuana in Alaska

Medical marijuana became legal in Alaska in 1999. With written approval from their physicians, patients can possess or transport up to 1 ounce of marijuana flower.

Under Alaska's law, approved conditions include:

Cachexia or Wasting Syndrome

Cancer

Chronic Pain

Glaucoma

HIV or AIDS

Multiple Sclerosis

Nausea

Seizures

Other conditions are subject to approval by the Alaska Department of Health and Social Services.

Consumption of CBD from Hemp Oil in Alaska

Hemp-derived CBD products are legal under Federal Law in the United States; however, individual state laws are dynamic and fluid. Individual states may enact their own laws governing hemp-derived CBD.

Cultivation of Cannabis in Alaska

Alaska's recreational marijuana law allows adults 21 and older to grow up to six plants on their personal properties, with up to one of the three plants mature at any one time. House Bill 75, which passed in July 2016, allows two adults 21 years of age or older that are residing in the same dwelling to grow up to 12 marijuana plants, which six or fewer being mature. Transportation of up to 6 immature plants is also legal, but all cannabis products

must be kept in the trunk of the car. Trimmings from these legally grown plants can be shared with adults over 21, but money cannot be exchanged.

Registered medical marijuana patients can grow up to six plants at home, although no more than three may be mature at any given time.

In 2018, Alaska passed a law to authorize the creation of a program to study the growth, cultivation and marketing of hemp and hemp-derived products like CBD.

Medical Marijuana in Arizona

In 2010, Arizona voters passed Proposition 203, legalizing the medical use of marijuana under the Arizona Medical Marijuana Act (AMMA). In order to use medical marijuana, you must be a qualifying patient who has registered with the Arizona Department of Health Services (ADHS) and received a registry identification card. To qualify as an Arizona medical marijuana patient, you must meet the follow criteria:

Be at least 18 years old

Have valid government-issued ID

Have Arizona residential address

Have medical records of past year and provide them to physician

Patient must have a "debilitating medical condition," which includes diseases such as:

Glaucoma

Cancer

HIV/AIDS

Post-traumatic stress disorder (PTSD)

Severe and chronic pain

Severe nausea

Getting a Medical Marijuana Card:

If you meet the above standards, the next step is to schedule an appointment with a doctor to obtain a Physician Certification Form. In addition to the cost of the doctor's visit, you will need to pay a $150 application fee to receive your card. Once you or your doctor's office submits your application, ADHS should mail your card to you within five business days. Note that you'll need to renew your card every year.

Out-of-State ID Card Reciprocity

If you're visiting Arizona and have a valid medical marijuana registration card from another state, you can possess and use marijuana in Arizona. However, you won't be able to get medical marijuana from an Arizona dispensary with an out-of-state ID card due to statutory limitations. No matter how much marijuana you're allowed in your home state, you can only possess and use up to 2.5 ounces of medical marijuana while in Arizona.

Where to Get Medical Marijuana

Patients with medical marijuana cards can obtain marijuana through dispensaries or growing their own, if approved by Arizona Department of Health Services to cultivate. If the nearest dispensary is 25 miles or more away from your residence, you can grow up to 12 plants.

Remember that qualifying patients can only purchase and possess 2.5 ounces of marijuana every two weeks. Additionally, medical marijuana cannot be smoked in public places, such as schools and parks. However, qualifying patients can consume marijuana in edible form in public places.

Cultivation

Under the Smart and Safe Marijuana act, Arizona residents over the age of 21 may grow up to 6 marijuana plants at their homes, if cultivation takes place within an enclosed area (such as a room, closet, or greenhouse) with a lock and is not visible from public view.

Marijuana patients can grow up to 12 plants of their own if they don't have a dispensary within 25 miles of their homes. Like recreational home cultivation, the plants have to be grown in an "enclosed, locked facility," which the law defines as a "closet, room, greenhouse, or other enclosed area equipped with locks or security devices that permit access only by a cardholder."

To grow with the law's blessing, you will also need the ADHS to designate you as a medical marijuana cultivator.

ADHS-designated caregivers can also grow and dispense medical marijuana for one to five medical marijuana patients. To be a caregiver, you have to be 21 years or older, agree to assist up to five medical marijuana patients, and have no previous drug felonies.

Medical Marijuana in Arkansas

With the support of 53 percent of voters, Arkansas passed Issue 6 in November 2016 to legalize medical marijuana. Issue 6, also known as the Arkansas Medical Marijuana Amendment, establishes a system for the cultivation, acquisition, and distribution of marijuana for qualifying patients. Patients must have a written certification from a licensed physician in the state to acquire access to cannabis for medical purposes. Home cultivation is not permitted.

In May 2019, two and a half years after Arkansans voted to legalize medical marijuana, the state's first dispensary opened its doors. The first dispensary to be officially licensed, located in Hot Springs, is the only one operating as of May 2019.

The following conditions have been approved under the law:

Alzheimer's Disease

Amyotrophic Lateral Sclerosis (ALS)

Cancer

Crohn's Disease

Fibromyalgia

Glaucoma

HIV/AIDS

Hepatitis C

Post-Traumatic Stress Disorder (PTSD)

Tourette's Syndrome

Severe Arthritis

Ulcerative Colitis

Additionally, medicinal cannabis can be recommended for any chronic or debilitating medical condition that produces:

Cachexia or Wasting Syndrome

Intractable Pain

Peripheral Neuropathy

Severe Nausea

Seizures

Severe and Persistent Muscle Spasms

The Department of Health can also approve medical marijuana for any other medical condition or its treatment.

Medical Marijuana in California

In 1996, California passed Proposition 215, making it the first state to legalize medical marijuana. Proposition 215, also known as the Compassionate Use Act of 1996 (Health & Safety Code, section 11362.5), was approved by 55.6% of voters and decriminalized the cultivation and use of medical marijuana by seriously ill individuals who receive a state-licensed physician's recommendation. Currently, a qualified patient or primary caregiver may possess no more than eight ounces of dried marijuana and maintain no more than six mature or 12 immature marijuana plants, unless they have a doctor's recommendation that this quantity does not meet their medical needs. The amount of marijuana that patients may possess and/or cultivate is also regulated locally and varies by city and county.

The California Department of Public Health established the Medical Marijuana Identification Card Program, a voluntary program which issues medical marijuana cards. In 2004, California's medical marijuana law was amended by Senate Bill

420, which added additional protections to the Compassionate Use Act. In 2015, the Medical Marijuana Regulation and Safety Act (which is comprised of three bills: AB 266, AB 243, and SB 643) was enacted to establish a licensing and regulatory framework for the cultivation, manufacture, transportation, storage, distribution, and sale of medical marijuana in California. The Medical Marijuana Regulation and Safety Act is expected to become fully implemented by January 1, 2018.

Ballot Proposition 215 received 56% 'yes' votes in November 1996, making California the very first state to legalize medical marijuana. Cannabis for medical purposes is legal for any patient with either a written or oral recommendation from a physician stating that they will benefit from medical marijuana. Medical marijuana cards can be acquired through the California Department of Public Health but are not required to purchase medical cannabis from a dispensary.

CALIFORNIA MEDICAL MARIJUANA STATISTICS AND FACTS

California defines medical cannabis as an agricultural product. The identification as an agricultural crop does not extend to other areas of the law. For example, cannabis is not an agricultural crop with respect to local "right to farm" ordinances.

Under California law, people who are entitled to use medical marijuana may also possess concentrated cannabis (hashish) for personal use. They may also produce concentrated cannabis but cannot use chemical solvents such as butane.

Currently, California law allows local governments to establish their own medical marijuana regulations.

California law allows local governments to pass ordinances imposing a tax on the cultivating, dispensing, producing, processing, preparing, storing, providing, donating, selling, or distributing of medical marijuana.

California jails don't have to accommodate medical marijuana use, but cannot prohibit an inmate from applying for a Medical Marijuana Identification Card.

Fifty-six of California's fifty-eight Counties participate in the Medical Marijuana Program (Colusa and Sutter County do not).

THE CALIFORNIA MEDICAL MARIJUANA IDENTIFICATION CARD PROGRAM

The California Department of Public Health's Medical Marijuana Identification Card Program

(MMICP) created a State-authorized Medical Marijuana ID Card and verification database to be used by law enforcement and the public. It verifies a patient or primary caregiver's authorization to possess, grow, transport, and/or use medical marijuana within California. Participation by patients and primary caregivers in the identification card program is voluntary. The verification website is located at http://mmic.cdph.ca.gov.here were 2,798 Medical Marijuana Program Cards issued in the Fiscal Year 2015-2016 (of which 884 were to Medi-Cal recipients).

HOW TO QUALIFY FOR A MEDICAL MARIJUANA CARD IN CALIFORNIA

You must be a have a valid California ID or a valid out-of-state ID or passport with proof of residency such as a lease agreement, utility bill, etc.

You must be 18 years of age or accompanied by a parent or guardian (unless you are lawfully emancipated, have declared self-sufficient minor status, or are a minor capable of medical consent)

You must obtain a medical marijuana recommendation from a state licensed physician stating that you have a serious medical condition and will benefit from the medicinal use of cannabis. Under the Medical Marijuana Program, a "serious medical condition" means all of the following:

Patients can possess up to 8 ounces of marijuana for any of the following conditions:

Anorexia

Arthritis

Cachexia or Wasting Syndrome

Cancer

Chronic Pain

Glaucoma

Severe nausea

HIV/AIDS

Migraine

Persistent Muscle Spasms, including those associated with Multiple Sclerosis

Seizures, including those associated with Epilepsy

California also allows medical marijuana for any chronic or persistent medical symptoms.

HOW TO APPLY FOR A MEDICAL MARIJUANA CARD IN CALIFORNIA

You will need to fill out an application, which can be downloaded here. You must reside in the California county where the application is submitted. You will need to provide the following current documentation with your application:

A copy of your doctor's recommendation

Proof of identity. This can be a valid California Department of Motor Vehicles (DMV) driver's license or valid identification (ID) card or another valid government-issued photo ID card

Proof of residency, which can be a:

Rent or mortgage agreement

Utility bill

California DMV motor vehicle registration

You must apply in person at your County's Program. There you will be asked to:

Pay the fee required by your County Program (Medi-Cal beneficiaries will receive a 50 percent reduction in the application fee)

Have your photo taken at the County Program's office. This photo will appear on your Medical Marijuana ID Card

FEES FOR A MEDICAL MARIJUANA CARD IN CALIFORNIA

The state fee for a Medical Marijuana Identification Card application is currently $66 per card (or $33 for Medi-Cal patients). Individual counties also have fees that vary by county. Please contact your County Program to find out what the total cost for a Medical Marijuana Identification Card is in your county.

CONTACT THE MEDICAL MARIJUANA PROGRAM

California Department of Public Health

Public Health Policy and Research Branch

Attention: Medical Marijuana Program Unit

MS 5202

P.O. Box 997377

Sacramento, CA 95899-7377

Telephone: (916) 552-8600

Fax: (916) 440-5591

Email: mmpinfo@cdph.ca.gov

MEDICAL MARIJUANA DISPENSARIES IN CALIFORNIA

California currently does not have a state-wide registry program for dispensaries, which are regulated at the city and county level. When the Medical Marijuana Regulation and Safety Act is fully implemented (expected to happen by January 01, 2018) the Department of Consumer Affairs' Bureau of Medical Marijuana Regulations will be responsible for regulating dispensaries. Meanwhile, dispensary owners are expected to obtain a Seller's Permit from the Board of Equalization and file Articles of Incorporation under the Corporations or Food and Agricultural Code. Also, depending on the local ordinances for the county or city the dispensary is located in, you may be required to obtain a business license and/or other permits.

CULTIVATION AND POSSESSION OF MEDICAL MARIJUANA IN CALIFORNIA

Under the Medical Marijuana Program, a qualified patient or primary caregiver may possess no more than eight ounces of dried marijuana and maintain no more than six mature or 12 immature marijuana plants. If a qualified patient or primary caregiver has a doctor's recommendation that this quantity does not meet the qualified patient's medical needs, the qualified patient or primary caregiver may possess an amount of marijuana consistent with the patient's needs. Counties and cities may retain or enact medical marijuana guidelines allowing qualified patients or primary caregivers to exceed these state limits.

Once the Medical Marijuana Regulation and Safety Act is fully implemented (which is expected to happen by January 01, 2018) the California Department of Food and Agriculture will regulate Medical Marijuana Cultivation.

THE MEDICAL MARIJUANA REGULATION AND SAFETY ACT (MMRSA)

Governor Brown signed the Medical Marijuana Regulation and Safety Act into law on October 09, 2015, and it became effective on January 01, 2016. The Act, composed of 3 bills (AB 266, AB 243, and SB 643) established a licensing and regulatory framework for the cultivation, manufacture, transportation, storage, distribution, and sale of medical cannabis in the State of California.

The Medical Marijuana Regulation and Safety Act established the Medical Cannabis Cultivation Program within the California Department of Food and Agriculture to license cultivators, establish conditions under which indoor and outdoor cultivation may occur, establish a track and trace program for reporting the movement of medical cannabis items through the distribution chain, and assist other state agencies in protecting the environment and public health.

Examples of requirements under the MMRSA include submission of fingerprint images to the Department of Justice, evidence of the legal right to occupy and use the proposed location as a cultivation site, submission of a detailed description of business operating procedures, and obtaining and maintaining a valid seller's permit.

REGULATORY AUTHORITIES ESTABLISHED BY THE MMRSA

The MMRSA tasks the following California Departments with establishing regulations for the medical cannabis industry:

Department of Food & Agriculture - Responsible for licensing cultivators and establishing a track and trace program through the Medical Cannabis Cultivation Program.

Department of Public Health - Responsible for licensing laboratories and manufacturers of products, such as edibles through the Office of Medical Cannabis Safety.

Department of Consumer Affairs -
Responsible for licensing transporters,
distributors, and dispensaries through the
Bureau of Medical Marijuana Regulations.

It is anticipated that licenses will begin
being issued under the Medical Marijuana
Regulation and Safety Act on Jan. 1, 2018.

THE THREE BILLS THAT COMPRISE
THE MMRSA (AB 266, AB 243, and SB
643)

Assembly Bill 266

Enacts the Medical Marijuana Regulation
and Safety Act for the licensure and
regulation of medical marijuana and
establishes within the Department of
Consumer Affairs the Bureau of Medical
Marijuana Regulation, under the supervision
and control of the Director of Consumer
Affairs.

Requires the Board of Equalization, in
consultation with the Department of Food
and Agriculture, to adopt a system for
reporting the movement of commercial
cannabis and cannabis products.

Imposes certain fines and civil penalties for
specified violations of the act and would

require moneys collected as a result of these fines and civil penalties to be deposited into the Medical Cannabis Fines and Penalties Account.

Provides that actions of licensees with the relevant local permits, in accordance with the act and applicable local ordinances, are not offenses subject to arrest, prosecution, or other sanction under State law.

Makes legislative findings to align with existing constitutional provisions that require that a statute that limits the right of access to the meetings of public bodies or the writings of public officials and agencies be adopted with findings demonstrating the interest protected by the limitation and the need for protecting that interest.

Read the Full Text of AB 266

Assembly Bill 243

Appropriates funds to implement the Medical Marijuana Regulation and Safety Act.

Requires the Department of Food and Agriculture, the Department of Pesticide Regulation, the State Department of Public Health, the Department of Fish and Wildlife, and the State Water Resources Control Board to promulgate regulations or standards relating to medical marijuana and its cultivation, as specified.

Requires various State agencies to take specified actions to mitigate the impact that marijuana cultivation has on the environment, and requires cities, counties, and their local law enforcement agencies to coordinate with State agencies to enforce laws addressing the environmental impacts of medical marijuana cultivation.

Requires a state licensing authority to charge each licensee under the Act licensure and renewal fees, as applicable, and deposit them into an account specific to that licensing authority in the Medical Marijuana and Safety Act Fund, which this bill creates. The bill also imposes certain fines and civil penalties for specified violations of the Medical Marijuana Regulation and Safety Act, and requires resulting moneys be deposited into the Medical Cannabis Fines and Penalties Account, also established by this bill within the fund.

Senate Bill 643

Sets forth standards for physicians and surgeons prescribing medical cannabis and requires the Medical Board of California to prioritize its investigative and prosecutorial resources to identify those who have repeatedly recommended excessive cannabis to patients for medical purposes or done so repeatedly without a good faith examination.

Requires applicants to furnish a full set of fingerprints in order to conduct criminal history record checks.

Requires, through the Medical Marijuana Regulation and Safety Act, that the Department of Food and Agriculture administer the provisions of the act related to and associated with the cultivation and transportation of medical cannabis. The Department of Food and Agriculture, in consultation with the Bureau, shall establish a track and trace program for reporting the movement of medical marijuana items throughout the distribution chain that utilizes a unique identifier. It also establishes State cultivator license types.

Requires the California Department of Public Health to oversee manufacturing and testing of medical cannabis.

Requires the Governor to appoint a chief, subject to Senate confirmation, of the

Bureau of Medical Marijuana Regulation, and requires the Department of Consumer Affairs to have the sole authority to create, issue, renew, discipline, suspend, or revoke licenses for the transportation and storage (unrelated to manufacturing) of medical marijuana, and would authorize the department to collect fees for its regulatory activities and impose related specified duties.

Authorizes counties to impose a tax on specified cannabis-related activity.

Medical Marijuana in Colorado

Medical marijuana has been legal in Colorado since 2001. With the written approval from a physician, patients can legally use, possess, and cultivate marijuana under the law.

Patients can possess up to 2 ounces of usable marijuana and up to 6 cannabis plants. They should always keep their doctor's documentation on hand to avoid arrest.

Colorado's medical marijuana law expands legal access to minors, provided they have parental consent. As of June 2016, schools in Colorado are required to allow students access to medical cannabis while on school grounds after Gov. John Hickenlooper signed "Jack's Law."

Approved conditions in Colorado are as follows:

Autism Spectrum Disorders

Cachexia or Wasting Syndrome

Cancer

Chronic Pain

Epilepsy and other Seizure Disorders

Glaucoma

HIV or AIDS

Multiple Sclerosis

Nausea

Opiate Replacement ("Any Condition for Which a Physician Could Prescribe an Opiate")

Post-Traumatic Stress Disorder (PTSD)

Other conditions are subject to approval by the Colorado Board of Health.

Consumption of CBD from Hemp Oil in Colorado.

Hemp-derived CBD products are legal under Federal Law in the United States; however, individual state laws are dynamic and fluid. Individual states may enact their own laws governing hemp-derived CBD.

Cultivation of Cannabis in Colorado

Colorado marijuana law allows individuals to grow up to six marijuana plants on their properties for both medical and non-medical purposes. However, just three of the plants can be mature at any one time. Trimmings from these plants can be shared with adults over 21 without financial remuneration.

The state has also legalized the cultivation of hemp by farmers licensed by the Colorado Department of Agriculture.

Medical Marijuana in Connecticut

Gov. Dannell Malloy signed into law House Bill 5389 in 2012 to legalize medical marijuana in Connecticut. Under the law, qualified patients can possess the amount that is 'reasonably necessary' for a one month's supply. Patients must always have their valid registration certificates on hand to avoid arrest, prosecution, and penalties.

Connecticut's medical marijuana program does have limitations as to who can be a qualified patient:

Must be a resident of Connecticut

Must not be an inmate

Must not be under the supervision of the Department of Corrections

If these conditions are not fulfilled, then individuals cannot possess, use, or cultivate medical marijuana regardless of their medical condition.

Medical marijuana can be sought for the following medical conditions:

Amyotrophic Lateral Sclerosis (ALS)

Cachexia or Wasting Syndrome

Cancer

Cerebral Palsy

Complex Regional Pain Syndrome

Crohn's Disease

Cystic Fibrosis

Epilepsy

Glaucoma

HIV or AIDS

Hydrocephalus with Intractable Headache

Interstitial Cystitis

Intractable Headache Syndromes

Intractable Neuropathic Pain

Intractable Spasticity

Irreversible Spinal Cord Injury with Objective Neurological Indication of Intractable Spasticity

Median Arcuate Ligament Syndrome (MALS)

Multiple Sclerosis (MS)

Muscular Dystrophy

Neuropathic Facial Pain

Osteogenesis Imperfecta (also called "Brittle Bone Disease")

Parkinson's Disease

Post Herpetic Neuralgia

Post Laminectomy Syndrome

Post-Surgical Back Pain with a condition called Chronic Radiculopathy

Post-Traumatic Stress Disorder (PTSD)

Severe Psoriasis and Psoriatic Arthritis

Severe Rheumatoid Arthritis

Sickle Cell Disease

Spasticity or Neuropathic Pain associated with Fibromyalgia

Terminal Illness Requiring End-Of-Life Care

Tourette Syndrome

Ulcerative Colitis

Uncontrolled Intractable Seizure Disorder

Vulvodynia and Vulvar Burning

Other medical approved by the Department
of Consumer Protection.

On May 17, 2016, Gov. Malloy signed
House Bill 5450, allowing patients under 18
to get legal access to medical marijuana. The
law went into effect on October 1, 2016.

Under the law, minors with a written
certification from two doctors and a written
statement of consent by a parent or guardian
can get legal access to medicinal cannabis
for:

Cerebral Palsy

Cystic Fibrosis

Epilepsy (Severe or Intractable)

Intractable Neuropathic Pain

Muscular Dystrophy

Osteogenesis imperfecta (also called "Brittle Bone
Disease")

Spinal Cord Injury (Irreversible)

Terminal Illness

Tourette Syndrome

The state's Medical Marijuana Program
Board of Physicians in September 2019

voted to add chronic pain and Ehrler-Danlos syndrome as qualifying conditions. The legislature's regulations review committee has final say whether the conditions will be added.

Consumption of CBD from Hemp Oil in Connecticut Hemp-derived CBD products are legal under Federal Law in the United States; however, individual state laws are dynamic and fluid. Individual states may enact their own laws governing hemp-derived CBD.

Cultivation of Cannabis in Connecticut

The cultivation of marijuana for medical or personal use is now allowed under Connecticut law.

The production of industrial hemp in Connecticut, however, is legal. In response to the legalization of hemp with the passage of the 2018 Farm Bill, Gov. Ned Lamont in May 2019 signed into law legislation that provides Connecticut farmers with an opportunity to "bolster their profits with hemp." The Connecticut Department of Agriculture must still establish its program and get it approved by the federal government. The new commercial hemp program will replace a research pilot program, put into place by Gov. Malloy in July 2015. The previous hemp law amended statues to allow institutions of higher education, or the state department of agriculture legalize to grow industrial hemp in Connecticut for research purposes.

Medical Marijuana in Delaware

The Delaware Medical Marijuana Act (Senate Bill 17), signed into law in 2011, legalized

Under the law, patients can possess up to 6 ounces of medical marijuana. They must register with only one compassion center, which cannot dispense more than 3 ounces of marijuana over a 14-day period.

Delaware's medical marijuana program has approved the following conditions:

Agitation of Alzheimer's Disease

Amyotrophic Lateral Sclerosis (ALS)

Autism with Aggressive or Self-Injurious Behavior

Cancer

Decompensated Cirrhosis

HIV/AIDS

Intractable Epilepsy

Multiple Sclerosis (MS)

Post-Traumatic Stress Disorder (PTSD)

Terminal Illness

A chronic or debilitating disease or medical condition or its treatments that producers one or more of the following:

Cachexia or Wasting Syndrome

Severe, Debilitating Pain

Intractable Nausea

Seizures

Severe and Persistent Muscle Spasms

Originally, the law required that patients need to be 18 and older, but in 2015 Gov. Jack Markell signed a bill that legalized marijuana based oils for minors under 18. Patients who are minors can only be recommended cannabis oil (CBD) containing no more than 7 percent THC, and/or oils containing 15 percent THC acid and no more than 7 percent THC.

The following conditions have been approved for minors:

Intractable Epilepsy

A chronic or debilitating disease or medical condition where they have failed treatment involving one or more of the following symptoms:

Cachexia or Wasting Syndrome

Intractable Nausea

Severe, Painful and Persistent Muscle Spasms

As of September 2016, qualified minors are legally allowed to use medicinal cannabis while on school grounds, thanks to the passing of Senate Bill 181, signed into law by Gov. Jack Markell.

District of Columbia Medical Marijuana

D.C. Law 23-128. Medical Marijuana Program Patient Employment Protection Temporary Amendment Act of 2020.

BE IT ENACTED BY THE COUNCIL OF THE DISTRICT OF COLUMBIA, that this act may be cited as the "Medical Marijuana Program Patient Employment Protection Temporary Amendment Act of 2020".

Sec. 2. The District of Columbia Government Comprehensive Merit Personnel Act of 1978, effective March 3, 1979 (D.C. Law 2-139; D.C. Official Code § 1-601.01 et seq.), is amended follows:

Note § 1-620.11

(a) Section 2051 (D.C. Official Code § 1-620.11) is amended as follows:

(1) Designate the existing text as subsection (a).

(2) A new subsection (b) is added to read as follows:

"(b) To the extent permitted by federal law and regulations, programs and rules adopted pursuant to subsection (a) of this section shall accommodate qualifying patients, as that term is defined in section 2(19) of the Legalization of Marijuana for Medical Treatment Initiative of 1999, effective July 27, 2010 (D.C. Law 18-210; D.C. Official Code § 7-1671.01(19)), in compliance with title XX-E.".

Note § 1-620.25

(b) Section 2025 (D.C. Official Code § 1-620.25) is amended by adding a new subsection (d) to read as follows:

"(d) Notwithstanding subsection (a) of this section, the testing program established pursuant to this title shall comply with the requirements of title XX-E.".

Note § 1-620.32

(c) Section 2032 (D.C. Official Code § 1-620.32) is amended by adding a new subsection (g) to read as follows:

"(g) The testing program established pursuant to this title shall comply with the requirements of title XX-E.".

Note § 1-620.44

(d) A new title XX-E is added to read as follows:

"TITLE XX-E. MEDICAL MARIJUANA
PROGRAM PATIENT EMPLOYMENT
PROTECTIONS.

"Sec. 2051. Definitions.

" For the purposes of this title, the term:

"(1) "Marijuana" shall have the same
meaning as provided in section 102(3)(A) of
the District of Columbia Uniform Controlled
Substances Act of 1981, effective August 5,
1981 (D.C. Law 4-29; D.C. Official Code §
48-901.02).

"(2) "Qualifying patient" shall have the
same meaning as provided in section 2(19)
of the Legalization of Marijuana for
Medical Treatment Initiative of 1999,
effective July 27, 2010 (D.C. Law 18-210;
D.C. Official Code § 7-1671.01(19)).

"(3) "Public employer" means the District
government.

"(4) "Safety sensitive position" means a
position with duties that, if performed while
under the influence of drugs or alcohol
could lead to a lapse of attention that could
cause actual, immediate, and permanent

physical injury or loss of life to self or others.

"Sec. 2052. Patient protections.

"(a)(1) Notwithstanding any other provision of law, except as provided in subsection (b) of this section, a public employer may not refuse to hire, terminate from employment, penalize, fail to promote, or otherwise take adverse employment action against an individual based upon the individual's status as a qualifying patient unless the individual used, possessed, or was impaired by marijuana at the individual's place of employment or during the hours of employment.

"(2) A qualifying patient's failure to pass a public employer-administered drug test for marijuana components or metabolites may not be used as a basis for employment-related decisions unless reasonable suspicion exists that the qualifying patient was impaired by marijuana at the qualifying patient's place of employment or during the hours of employment.

"(b) Subsection (a) of this section shall not apply to safety sensitive positions or if compliance would cause the public employer to commit a violation of a federal law, regulation, contract, or funding agreement.".

Note § 24-211.22

Sec. 3. Section 3 of the Department of Corrections Employee Mandatory Drug and Alcohol Testing Act of 1996, effective September 20, 1996 (D.C. Law 11-158; D.C. Official Code § 24-211.22), is amended by adding a new subsection (d) to read as follows:

"(d) The testing program established pursuant to this act shall comply with the requirements of title XX-E of the District of Columbia Government Comprehensive Merit Personnel Act of 1978, passed on 2nd reading June 9, 2020 (Enrolled version of Bill 23-756).".

Sec. 4. Fiscal impact statement.

The Council adopts the fiscal impact statement of the Budget Director as the fiscal impact statement required by section 4a of the General Legislative Procedures Act of 1975, approved October 16, 2006 (120 Stat. 2038; D.C. Official Code § 1-301.47a).

Sec. 5. Effective date.

(a) This act shall take effect following approval by the mayor (or in the event of veto by the mayor, action by the Council to override the veto), a 30-day period of congressional review as provided in section 602(c)(1) of the District of Columbia Home Rule Act, approved December 24, 1973 (87 Stat. 813; D.C. Official Code § 1-206.02(c)(1)), and publication in the District of Columbia Register.

(b) This act shall expire after 225 days of its having taken effect.

QUALIFYING CONDITIONS:

Any debilitating condition as recommended by a DC licensed doctor

PATIENT POSSESSION LIMITS:

Two ounces

HOME CULTIVATION:

No

STATE-LICENSED DISPENSARIES ALLOWED:

Yes, medical dispensaries may grow up to
500 plants on site at any one time. Both non-
profit and for-profit organizations are
eligible to operate the dispensaries.

STATE-LICENSED DISPENSARIES
OPERATIONAL:

Yes

MEDICAL MARIJUANA STATUTES:

D.C. Act 13-138 §2 (3) (2010)

CAREGIVERS:

Yes, a caregiver is a person designated by a
qualifying patient as the person authorized
to possess, obtain from a dispensary,
dispense, and assist in the administration of
medical marijuana. The caregiver must be
18 years of age or older. The caregiver must
be registered with the Department as the
qualifying patient's caregiver. A caregiver
may only serve one qualifying patient at a
time.

ESTIMATED NUMBER OF REGISTERED
PATIENTS:

6,309

Source: Department of Health, Health Regulation and Licensing Administration:

RECIPROCITY:

Yes. Separate legislation approved by the Council in 2017 "provides access to medical marijuana in the District of Columbia to those patients enrolled in a medical marijuana program from other jurisdictions."

Medical Marijuana in Florida

Florida had a very restrictive high-CBD, low-THC marijuana law for a couple of years before 71% of voters approved Amendment 2 in November 2016 to allow full medical cannabis. Amendment 2 went into effect January 3, 2017, and the Florida Legislature passed legislation that implemented the amendment in July 2017.

Under Florida's Right to Medical Marijuana Initiative, patients suffering from debilitating medical conditions are allowed medical use of marijuana provided they have a doctor's recommendation and an identification card. Home cultivation for medical purposes is not permitted under the law. The law does allow qualifying patients to have a caregiver who is at least 21 years old to assist in the collection and administering of medical cannabis.

Originally, Florida marijuana laws permitted only medical cannabis oils, sprays, tinctures, edibles, and vaping materials. While smoking marijuana was originally not permitted under the law, in 2018 Leon County Circuit Judge Karen Gievers ruled that the constitutional amendment approved by Florida voters in 2016 broadly legalized medical marijuana and gave eligible patients the right to smoke marijuana in private. In March 2019, the Florida Legislature approved SB 182, a bill that overturns the ban on smokable forms of medical marijuana for adults and patients under 18 who are either diagnosed with a terminal illness or who have obtained a second recommendation from a pediatrician.

SB 182 also allows patients to order a 210-day supply of medical marijuana at a time, up from the original 70-day supply limit approved in the initial legislation.

Who Can Be Treated with Medical Marijuana Under Florida Marijuana Laws?

Florida's medical marijuana program allows medical marijuana to be provided as treatment for patients with the following "debilitating medical conditions":

Amyotrophic Lateral Sclerosis (ALS)

Cancer

Crohn's disease

Epilepsy

Glaucoma

HIV/AIDS

Multiple sclerosis

Parkinson's disease

Post-traumatic stress disorder (PTSD)

"Other debilitating medical conditions of the same kind or class as or comparable to those enumerated."

Additionally, in June 2019, Gov. Ron DeSantis signed into law HB 7107 to allow a cannabis-derived drug for children with epilepsy. The bill changes that specific drug's classification in state law from a Schedule I substance to Schedule V.

Senate Bill 862, signed into law by Gov. Ben Cayetano in 2000, legalized marijuana for medical purposes. Provided a patient has a written certification from a physician, the use and possession of up to 4 ounces of usable marijuana and no more than 7 marijuana plants (up to 3 mature marijuana plants, 4 immature marijuana plants) is legal under the law.

Qualifying patients are allowed to have a primary caregiver, who is a person 18 years of age or older that is responsible for managing the well-being of the qualifying patient with respect to medical marijuana.

The following conditions have been approved conditions for medical marijuana possession:

Amyotrophic Lateral Sclerosis (ALS)

Alzheimer's Disease

Cachexia or Wasting Syndrome

Cancer

Crohn's Disease

Glaucoma

Hepatitis C

HIV/AIDS

Post-Traumatic Stress Disorder (PTSD)

Seizures (including Epilepsy)

Severe and Chronic Pain

Severe or Persistent Muscle Spasms (including Multiple Sclerosis)

Severe Nausea

In-State (Hawaii) & Out of State Registered patients and caregivers are prohibited from acquiring, possessing, cultivating, using, distributing or transporting cannabis or paraphernalia in ALL public places. This includes (but not limited to):

Public Parks and Beaches

Recreation Centers, Youth Centers

School Grounds

In a moving vehicle including school buses or public buses

In the workplace of one's employment

In addition, Act 241 amended part IX HRS HRS-329– 122 in that cannabis:

"…shall be transported in a sealed container, not be visible to the public, and shall not be removed from it sealed container or consumed or used in any way while it is in the public place"; and

"…transport does not include the inter-island transportation of cannabis, usable cannabis, or any manufactured cannabis product". This means that registered patients and caregivers CANNOT transport cannabis inter-island.

Hotels, Apartments, and Condos

A general rule of thumb – if the entire "footprint" of the property is "smoke free", registered in-state and out-of-state patients cannot smoke or ingest via safe pulmonary device (a.k.a. vape) medical cannabis anywhere on that property.

There are other methods of ingestion.

The smell of cannabis smoke from a neighbor's home/hotel room (single family, condo, hotel, etc.) – again, all "smoke free" laws apply to medical cannabis.

Registry staff refer complainants to their Board of Directors or property managers (for condos/apartments) or to speak directly to their neighbors in this regard.

Owner's or tenants should be able to obtain a copy of the By-Laws from their Board of Directors.

The smell of cannabis plants growing in a neighbor's yard – there is currently no legal guidance in this regard.

Registry staff typically recommend that the complainant file a report with local law enforcement to verify if the site is appropriately registered and/or speak directly with their neighbor in this regard.

Other smells or questionable activity from a neighbor's home –

Registry staff typically recommend that the complainant file a report with the Narcotics Enforcement Division to rule out other illicit activities.

Note: Patients should always keep their medical marijuana certification on hand to avoid any trouble with the law.

Illinois Medical Marijuana

Illinois was the twentieth state to legalize medical marijuana on January 1, 2014. Known as The Compassionate Use of Medical Cannabis Act, this program is still in a pilot stage and was recently extended until at least July 2020. Illinois' medical program was also expanded by the CRTA, allowing medical patients to cultivate in their homes.

Possession:

As of January 1, 2020, Illinois residents 21 and older may possess 30 grams of cannabis flower, 500 mg of THC-infused edible products (amount is cumulative, regardless of being in a single product or multiple products), or five grams of concentrate. Non-residents to Illinois may purchase 15 grams of cannabis, 250 mg of THC in a cannabis-infused product, or 2.5 grams of concentrated cannabis product.

Qualifying patients are able to possess an "adequate supply" of medical marijuana. An adequate supply refers to 2.5 ounces of usable cannabis. However, patients may apply for a waiver to possess more than the

2.5-ounce limit based on the treatment required for their debilitating medical condition(s).

Purchasing Limits:

Recreational purchasing limits are capped at 30 grams of cannabis flower or its equivalent in other forms of marijuana products.

On the medical side of things, in order to purchase medical marijuana, a qualifying patient must register and possess a valid registry identification card by the Department of Public Health. Qualifying patients are allowed to purchase an "adequate supply" of medical marijuana. The standard measurement of an adequate supply is 2.5 ounces every 14 days. A patient may apply for a waiver to purchase more than 2.5 ounces if a physician provides a signed, written statement confirming that 2.5 ounces is insufficient as an adequate supply to alleviate a debilitating medical condition. When purchasing concentrates, edibles or other marijuana products that are not flower, the pre-weight of the marijuana flower used to make the product is added towards the purchase limit.

Qualifying Patients:

Under Illinois law, a qualifying patient is a person diagnosed by a licensed physician as having a debilitating medical condition. Current accepted debilitating medical conditions are listed as follows:

ALS

Alzheimer's Disease

Arachnoiditis

Arnold-Chiari Malformation

Cachexia/Wasting Syndrome

Cancer

Causalgia

CIDP

Crohn's Disease

CRPS

Dystonia

Fibrous Dysplasia

Glaucoma

Hepatitis C

HIV/AIDS

Hydrocephalus

Hydromyelua

Interstitial Cystitis

Lupus

Multiple Sclerosis

Muscular Dystrophy

Myasthenia Gravis

Myoclonus

Nail-Patella Syndrome

Neurofibromatosis

Parkinson's

PTSD

Reflex Sympathetic Dystrophy

Residual Limb Pain

Rheumatoid Arthritis

RSD

Seizures

Severe Fibromyalgia

Sjorgen's Syndrome

Spinal Cord Injury

Spinocerebellar Ataxia

Syringomyelia

Tarlov Cysts

Terminal Illness (< 6 months)

Tourette's

Traumatic Brain Injury

Consumption:

Adults 21 years of age and older are legally able to consume cannabis purchased from licensed dispensaries. Public cannabis consumption is illegal and strictly prohibited. Other restrictions apply as well. Cannabis consumption is also prohibited in:

Any motor vehicle:

On school grounds (with exception for approved medical patients)

Any place near someone under the age of 21

Any place near an on-duty school bus driver, police officer, firefighter or corrections officer

Landlords, employers, private clubs and universities will all be allowed to prohibit cannabis use as well.

Only adults 21 years of age or older and qualifying patients with a valid registry identification card are able to consume cannabis products in Illinois. It is illegal for any person who is under 21 years of age and not a qualified patient to consume cannabis.

Driving Under the Influence:

Driving under the influence of cannabis is illegal and strictly prohibited. Those caught behind the wheel under the influence of marijuana face steep charges in the same fashion of an alcohol DUI. In addition to driving a motor vehicle under the influence of cannabis, it is also illegal to operate an aircraft, motorboat or any other motor vehicle while under the influence of cannabis.

Transporting Marijuana:

It is illegal to transport marijuana in car unless it is in a secured, sealed and tamper-evident container that is inaccessible while the vehicle is moving. The vehicle must also be private and not open to the public. Under no circumstance is it legal for a driver or passenger to consume recreational or medical cannabis inside of a vehicle.

Exporting Marijuana:

It is illegal to export marijuana from Illinois and those who are caught doing face severe penalties. It is not worth the risk, so be sure to only consume cannabis products lawfully and never export it over state lines.

Cultivation:

Under Illinois' new recreational cannabis laws, it is illegal for adults to grow their own cannabis. All recreational cannabis must be legally purchased at a licensed dispensary.

Beginning on January 1, 2020, medical cannabis patients may grow up to five plants at their residence, with a limit of five plants per household, regardless of the number of patients residing in the house. Patients may purchase cannabis seeds from a dispensary and any plants in a residence must be secured. Harvests cultivated from home grows will not violate the medical patient's possession limit, however, the cannabis must be stored within the residence, and outside possession limits still apply in public.

Medical Marijuana in Louisiana

The Louisiana State Legislature signed SB 143 into law in June 2015 to lay the framework for medicinal marijuana access, but regulatory hurdles have caused the program's launch to be delayed. To try to kick-start the program, Gov. John Bel Edwards signed a bill in May 2016 that expands the program to include more conditions and allows doctors to "recommend" rather than "prescribe" marijuana to patients.

Medical marijuana in Louisiana became available to patients starting in August 2019. Agricultural centers at Louisiana State University and Southern University have been selected to grow cannabis for the state, overseen by the state agriculture department. Nine dispensaries have been selected throughout the state.

Medical marijuana will be allowed in the form of medicinal oils, pills, liquids, and topical applications. In June 2019, Louisiana lawmakers passed a bill allowing for the sale and use of cannabis inhalers.

When Can a Doctor Recommend Medical Marijuana in Louisiana?

Despite launch delays, lawmakers have continued to make efforts to improve the program. In June 2018, Gov. Edwards signed into law two measures that expand the state's medical marijuana program. House Bill 579 added glaucoma, severe muscle spasms, intractable pain, post-traumatic stress disorder (PTSD), and Parkinson's disease as qualifying conditions. House Bill 672 allows for medical marijuana to be used in the treatment of autism spectrum disorder.

A full list of the conditions that are approved for medical marijuana under Louisiana law is as follows:

Autism

Cachexia or wasting syndrome

Cancer

Crohn's disease

Epilepsy

Glaucoma

HIV/AIDS

Intractable pain

Multiple sclerosis

Muscular dystrophy

Parkinson's disease

Post-traumatic stress disorder (PTSD)

Seizure disorders

Severe muscle spasms

Spasticity

Tax Stamps Required on Medical Marijuana:

Tax stamps are another unique aspect of Louisiana marijuana laws. In short, licensed sellers of medical marijuana are required to place a state-issued stamp on marijuana packaging and containers. These stamps not only require distributors to clearly mark any marijuana products they have on them, but it also helps the state collect taxes on the sale of medical marijuana.

Tax stamps cost $3.50 per gram of marijuana if the owner is in possession of 42.5 grams of marijuana or more. If an individual is caught with cannabis that does not have a tax stamp, they are subject to a fine that is 200% the cost of the original tax stamps, as well as the possibility of up to five years in prison.

Medical Marijuana Prohibited Locations in Louisiana:

A drug-free zone is a designated area in Louisiana in which no controlled substances can be present, no matter the circumstances. This includes both recreational and medical marijuana, and possession or use can be charged with violating a drug-free zone, even if you have a medical marijuana license. Drug-free zones include elementary and high schools, universities and colleges, religious buildings such as churches or temples, childcare facilities, public housing, and drug treatment facilities.

Not only are you not allowed to have drugs directly in these zones, but you are not allowed to have drugs within 2,000 feet of drug-free zones. If you are caught possessing, distributing, or cultivating marijuana within 2,000 feet of a drug-free zone, any penalties will be punishable by 1.5 times the maximum sentence. That means that if you are caught in possession of 14 grams or less of marijuana, you may be

subject to a $450 fine and 22 days in jail, as
that is 1.5 times the standard $300 fine and a
15-day jail sentence.

Medical Marijuana in Maine

Medical marijuana was legalized in Maine on November 2, 1999, when more than 60 percent of voters approved the Maine Medical Use of Marijuana Act. Under the law, qualified patients or caregivers can carry up to 2.5 ounces of medical marijuana and cultivate up to 6 mature marijuana plants. A primary caregiver must be 21 years or older and should have no prior disqualifying drug offenses.

Under Maine marijuana laws, visitors who have valid registry identification cards to use medical marijuana from other states are allowed to use medical cannabis for 30 days without having to obtain a Maine registry identification card. Visitors, however, are not permitted to purchase medical marijuana in Maine.

Maine has awarded licenses to 8 dispensaries that are now fully operational.

Cultivation of Cannabis in Maine:

The cultivation of up to 6 flowering marijuana plants and 12 immature marijuana plants by adults 21 and older is legal under

Maine's Question 1. The law also allows adults to cultivate unlimited seedlings.

Registered medical marijuana patients and caregivers can grow up to 6 marijuana plants, out of which only 3 may be mature at one time. If a patient has named 2 primary caregivers, only of them can cultivate medical marijuana.

Individuals in Maine can also apply for federal permits to cultivate industrial hemp under the LD 1159 Act of 2009.

Approved conditions are as follows:

Alzheimer's Disease

Amyotrophic Lateral Sclerosis (ALS)

Cachexia or Wasting Syndrome

Cancer

Chronic Pain

Crohn's Disease

Epilepsy

Glaucoma

Hepatitis C

HIV/AIDS

Huntington's Disease

Inflammatory Bowel Disease

Multiple Sclerosis (MS)

Nail-patella Syndrome

Nausea

Parkinson's Disease

Post-Traumatic Stress Disorder (PTSD)

Medical Marijuana in Maryland

Medical marijuana was legalized in Maryland in 2014 when House Bill 881 was signed into law. Patients must acquire a written certification from a licensed physician and register with the state's program. Under the law, children who meet their physician's criteria for treatment can become legal patients in Maryland. The Maryland Medical Cannabis Commission (MMCC) and the Maryland Department of Health and Mental Hygiene are responsible for developing regulations for marijuana access.

Qualified patients can possess up to 120 grams, or approximately four ounces, at one time, unless a physician makes a special determination that a patient needs more. Medical cannabis is available in forms that can be vaporized (not smoked), or extracts, lotions, ointments, and tinctures.

The law approves the following conditions for medical marijuana:

Anorexia

Cachexia or Wasting Syndrome

Glaucoma

Post-Traumatic Stress Disorder (PTSD)

Seizures

Severe or Chronic Pain

Severe Loss of Appetite

Severe Nausea

Severe or Persistent Muscle Spasms

Any condition that is severe, for which other medical treatments have been ineffective.

The cultivation of marijuana for personal or medical use is illegal in Maryland and may only be done by licensed growers. In April 2016, Governor Larry Hogan signed House Bill 443, which permits the Department of Agriculture to authorize institutions of higher education to grow hemp for academic research. Legislators then established the Maryland Industrial Hemp Research Pilot Program after passing House Bill 698, which took effect July 2018.

Medical Marijuana in Massachusetts

Residents of Massachusetts can legally purchase cannabis from state-licensed dispensaries. All cannabis products, both medical and recreational, must be consumed on private property as public consumption of marijuana, even medical marijuana is still illegal. This includes smoking, vaping, or consumption of edibles. Marijuana can't be smoked where tobacco smoking is banned.

The Department of Public Health (DPH) advises all commercial cannabis growers to test their harvested crops as well as all marijuana products for safety, quality, and potency. Certified labs must analyze the following: cannabinoid makeup and potency, fungal mycotoxins, residual solvents, pesticides, plant growth regulators, and microbiological contaminants.

Qualifying Conditions:

Amyotrophic lateral sclerosis (ALS)

Cancer

Crohn's disease

Glaucoma

Hepatitis C

HIV/AIDS

Multiple sclerosis (MS)

Medical Marijuana in Michigan

Proposition 1 signed into law in November 2018, allows adults in Michigan to purchase and possess up to 2.5 ounces of cannabis legally in public and grow up to 12 plants at home, out of plain sight. Medical cannabis is also available in state-licensed dispensaries.

Cannabis manufacturers are required by the Michigan Medical Marijuana Program (MMMP) to send its products to cannabis testing labs also known as "safety compliance labs." These laboratories must test for the following: THC and THCA levels, CBD and CBDA levels, terpenes, chemical residue, pesticides, fungicides, insecticides, herbicides, mycotoxin, and water content.

Qualifying Conditions & Patient Rights

Alzheimer's disease

Amyotrophic lateral sclerosis (ALS)

Arthritis

Autism

Cancer

Chronic pain

Colitis/ulcerative colitis

Crohn's disease

Glaucoma

Hepatitis C

HIV/AIDS

Inflammatory bowel disease

Nail patella,

Obsessive-compulsive disorder

Parkinson's disease

Post-traumatic stress disorder (PTSD)

Rheumatoid arthritis

Spinal cord injury

Tourette syndrome

Or the treatment of the following conditions:

A chronic or debilitating disease or medical condition or its treatment that results in wasting syndrome

Seizures

Severe and chronic pain

Severe and persistent muscle spasms.

Severe nausea

Medical Marijuana Law in Minnesota

Residents may possess Usable Marijuana: a maximum of a 30-day supply of the dosage determined for that patient. Pharmacists at registered Cannabis Patient Centers recommend specific dosage and type for patients.

Cancer (if the underlying condition or treatment produces severe or chronic pain, nausea or severe vomiting, or cachexia or severe wasting),

Qualifying Conditions:

Glaucoma,

HIV/AIDS,

Tourette's syndrome,

ALS,

Seizures/epilepsy,

Severe and persistent muscle spasms/MS,

Crohn's disease,

Terminal illness with a life expectancy of under one year, PTSD,

Intractable pain; Chronic pain,

Age-related macular degeneration,

Autism spectrum disorders,

Obstructive sleep apnea.

Medical Marijuana law in Mississippi

Medical marijuana is legal in Mississippi. Recreational use is prohibited. Mississippi enacted medical legalization in 2020.

The penalties for marijuana in Mississippi are among the most severe in the U.S. and can include a minimum 2 years in jail for growing a single plant.

Possession of less than 30 grams is a maximum $250 fine, but you're looking at a minimum one to two years in prison for a single THC vape cart bought out of state.

Mississippi has about 5,000 marijuana arrests per year.

Mississippi voters legalized medical cannabis on Nov. 3, 2020, with Initiative 65. A dominating 74% of voters approved the measure.

The Medical Marijuana 2020 campaign gathered 228,000 signatures to place Initiative 65 on the ballot.

Initiative 65 legalizes up to 2.5 ounces of cannabis every 14 days, if bought from a "marijuana treatment center" that is licensed by the state. There's a $100 fine for smoking medical weed in public.

Qualifying debilitating conditions that would make you eligible for a medical marijuana card in Mississippi:

Cancer

Epilepsy or other seizures

Parkinson's disease

Huntington's disease

Muscular dystrophy

Multiple sclerosis

Cachexia

Post-traumatic stress disorder (PTSD)

Positive status for human immunodeficiency virus

Acquired immune deficiency syndrome

Chronic or debilitating pain

Amyotrophic lateral sclerosis

Glaucoma

Agitation of dementias

Crohn's disease

Ulcerative colitis

Sickle-cell anemia

Autism with aggressive or self-injurious behaviors

Pain refractory to appropriate opioid management

Spinal cord disease or severe injury

Intractable nausea

Severe muscle spasticity

After an in-person exam, a state-licensed doctor would write you a "physician certificate" good for 12 months or shorter. Minors would need a parent or guardian. A physician's certificate gets you a state medical marijuana card, which is good at the treatment centers.

Are edibles legal in Mississippi?

Edibles like pot brownies, gummies, and hard candy are very much not legal and come with severe jail time, based on the weight of the brownies, not the weight of the THC inside.

CBD is legal in Mississippi, so long as the plant or product it is in has under 0.3% THC.

In 2020, Mississippi followed federal changes and legalized hemp with the Mississippi Hemp Cultivation Act, including licensing and regulation.

The program's roll-out is pending a state plan and could be slowed by federal regulation at the USDA. The Act removes hemp from the state's Controlled Substances schedule.

Medical Marijuana Law in Missouri

Medical cannabis is legal in Missouri, but recreational cannabis use is not.

In 2018, Missourians passed Amendment 2 for the medical use of marijuana in the state, and in late 2019 and early 2020, the state began awarding licenses to dispensaries, labs, cultivators, and producers. Sales to medical marijuana program participants slowly rolled out as dispensaries opened.

The Missouri Department of Health and Senior Services oversees the medical marijuana program for the state, including applications and licensing for businesses, patients, and caregivers.

It costs $25 for patients and caregivers to apply for medical marijuana and $100 for a patient cultivation license.

You are not allowed to grow marijuana in Missouri unless you have a medical marijuana license as a patient cultivator.

Medical marijuana patients are allowed to grow up to six plants after paying an additional fee with their medical marijuana license to be a patient cultivator.

There are also rules about shared cultivation. This means that, in the state of Missouri, a maximum of two individuals may cultivate in the same space. This can include two patients, two caregivers, or any combination of the licensed two.

Qualifying conditions for medical marijuana in Missouri must be approved by an MD or OD licensed to practice in Missouri.

Cancer

Epilepsy

Glaucoma

Intractable migraines unresponsive to other treatment

A chronic medical condition that causes severe, persistent pain or persistent muscle spasms, including but not limited to those associated with multiple sclerosis, seizures, Parkinson's disease, and Tourette's syndrome.

A debilitating psychiatric disorder, including, but not limited to, post-traumatic stress order if diagnosed by a state-licensed psychiatrist.

Human immunodeficiency virus or acquired immune deficiency syndrome

A chronic medical condition that is normally treated with a prescription medication that could lead to physical or psychological dependence, when a physician determines that medical use of marijuana could be effective in treating that condition and would serve as a safer alternative to the prescription medication.

A terminal illness

In the professional judgment of a physician, any other chronic, debilitating, or other medical condition, including, but not limited to, hepatitis C, amyotrophic lateral sclerosis (ALS), inflammatory bowel disease, Crohn's disease, Huntington's disease, autism, neuropathies, sickle cell anemia, agitation of Alzheimer's disease, cachexia, and wasting syndrome.

Medical Marijuana Law in Montana

Montana's medical marijuana program has been riddled with setbacks and resets since it was first passed into law in 2004. After an initial explosion of dispensaries and years of what state officials characterized as "minimal oversight," federal authorities began raiding Montana's dispensaries. In 2011, the state Legislature approved a measure that limited dispensaries to serving no more than three total patients.

Implementation of that law was delayed by years of court challenges, and it finally took effect in 2016, effectively removing 93% of Montana's medical cannabis patients off the state program and into the illicit market.

But later that year, voters approved a new statewide measure that repealed the three-patient rule. It took nearly three years for the program to return its patient base to pre-2011 levels.

Currently, about 38,000 Montanans have state-issued medical marijuana cards. To be registered as a medical marijuana patient in Montana, a physician may recommend the use of medical marijuana.

The following conditions qualify for treatment with medical marijuana if approved by attending physician.

Cancer, glaucoma, or positive status for human immunodeficiency virus, or acquired immune deficiency syndrome when the condition or disease results in symptoms that seriously and adversely affect the patient's health status

Cachexia or wasting syndrome

Severe chronic pain that is persistent pain of severe intensity that significantly interferes with daily activities as documented by the patient's treating physician.

Intractable nausea or vomiting

epilepsy or an intractable seizure disorder

Multiple sclerosis

Crohn's disease

Painful peripheral neuropathy

A central nervous system disorder resulting in chronic, painful spasticity or muscle spasms

Admittance into hospice care

Post-traumatic stress disorder (PTSD)

Medical Marijuana Law in Nevada

Patients, caregivers, and adults 21 and older can purchase and consume cannabis from licensed retailers or a Nevada dispensary. Recreational users pay a 10% excise tax. No one is allowed to purchase more than 1 ounce of cannabis at a time.

Jurisdiction over both the medical marijuana and adult-use programs belongs to the Nevada Department of Taxation. while the Division of Public and Behavioral Health (DPBH) currently administers the Medical Marijuana Patient Cardholder Registry.

It is illegal to consume cannabis in any public space in Nevada, therefore consumption must take place on private property, if the property owner has not prohibited it. Cannabis may not be used in any moving vehicle by the driver or passenger, and it is illegal to drive under the influence of marijuana.

Medical marijuana patients and caregivers can possess up to 2.5 ounces of edibles, flower, concentrates, or topicals per two-week period. Patients may grow up to 12 plants for medical purposes.

All patients who qualify for the program
must have a recommendation from a
certified physician in order to obtain medical
marijuana with a Nevada marijuana license.
Only patients who have been diagnosed with
a chronic or debilitating medical condition
in which the medical use of marijuana may
mitigate the symptoms or effects of that
condition will receive recommendations and
will be issued a registry card.

Addiction to opioids

Anorexia

Anxiety disorder

Autism

Autoimmune disease

Cancer

Cachexia, or wasting syndrome

Glaucoma

HIV/AIDS

Neuropathic conditions

Persistent muscle spasms, including those
caused by multiple sclerosis

Seizures, including those caused by epilepsy and Severe nausea or pain

 Any other chronic or debilitating medical condition as classified by the DPBH, or upon the acceptance of a petition to add a condition to Nevada's recognized list of conditions. Patients in the registry who require assistance obtaining or using medical cannabis may only designate one caregiver. Caregivers must be at least 18 years old and a permanent resident of Nevada. Caregivers must be designated as a primary caregiver by the patient and can only provide care for one patient at a time. They must also be the primary person who's responsible for the person diagnosed with a chronic or debilitating medical condition. Approved caregivers can pick up their patients' medical cannabis at a designated dispensary, and can possess, transport, and administer a patient's medical marijuana after purchase. Caregivers cannot be medical cannabis users themselves.

Dispensaries are authorized to sell to out-of-state medical marijuana patients who have medical marijuana cards from their home state.

All cannabis grown and processed in Nevada must be tested by an independent testing laboratory. Laboratories must receive a medical marijuana establishment registration certificate before performing any cannabis quality assurance test. Subsequently, labs must meet certain criteria in order to complete the certification process to conduct tests.

Labs must analyze for the following:

Cannabinoids

Foreign matter

Heavy metals

Microbes

Moisture content

Pesticide and other toxic chemical residue

Potency

Solvents

Terpenes

Medical Marijuana Law in New Hampshire

Medical marijuana may be purchased at a licensed dispensary storefront but cannot be consumed in public. Nor are there delivery services in the either.

Each batch of cannabis grown within an Alternative Treatment Center (ATC) should be tested for its cannabinoid profile. Cannabinoids to be tested include THC, THCV, CBC, CBD, CBN, and CBG. These tests must be completed at an accredited testing lab. Water and soil tests also required.

Multiple Sclerosis,

Chronic pancreatitis,

Spinal cord injury or disease,

Traumatic brain injury,

Epilepsy,

Lupus,

Parkinson's disease,

Alzheimer's disease,

Or one or more injuries that significantly interferes with daily activities as documented by the patient's provider, or a severely debilitating or terminal medical condition or its treatment that has produced at least one of the following:

Elevated intraocular pressure,

Cachexia,

Chemotherapy-induced anorexia,

Wasting syndrome,

Agitation of Alzheimer's disease,

Severe pain that has not responded to previously prescribed medication or surgical measures or for which other treatment options produced serious side effects, constant or severe nausea, moderate to severe vomiting, seizures, or severe, persistent muscle spasms.

Patients in New Hampshire may possess 2oz. of flower or concentrate.

Medical Marijuana Law in New Jersey

Adults 18 and older may purchase and possess 2 oz. of medical marijuana from Alternative Treatment Centers (ATCs), if patients have a physician's recommendation. Medical patients pay 4% in sales tax though it's set to be eliminated in July 2022. New Jersey medical marijuana patients may only consume cannabis in the privacy of their homes. Smoking medical marijuana falls under the same regulations as tobacco smoking in the Smoke-Free Air Act.

The New Jersey Department of Health (HJDOH) must collect soil and plant samples, as well as samples of any product containing cannabis that is cultivated or sold by a medical marijuana dispensary or ATC. This testing process is to ensure quality control and safety for qualifying medical cannabis patients.

New Jersey patients holding a medical marijuana card may possess 2 oz. of flower or concentrates within a 30-day period.

Under certain circumstances, a patient may receive instructions authorizing a 90-day supply of medical marijuana, as per N.J.R.S. §24:6I-10. To do so, the patient must have multiple written instructions from their physician, since each written instruction is valid for only a 30-day period. Additionally, the patient must satisfy the following conditions:

Each set of written instructions is for a "legitimate medical purpose"

Each set of instructions indicates the earliest date on which the patient may receive the medical marijuana

Their physician has determined that obtaining a 90-day supply does not create an undue risk of abuse.

As of September 14, 2020, Amyotrophic lateral sclerosis (ALS), or Lou Gehrig's disease

Anxiety Cachexia, or wasting syndrome

Chronic pain related to musculoskeletal disorders

Chronic pain in the Internal organs, Abdomen, or intestines

HIV/AIDS Inflammatory bowel disease, including Crohn's disease

Migraines

Dystrophy Multiple sclerosis

Nausea and vomiting Tourette's syndrome

Terminal cancer or illness were qualifying
conditions.

If the physician determines the patient has
less than 12 months to live

Opioid addiction Patients will also qualify if they
are resistant to conventional therapy for:

Glaucoma Intractable skeletal muscular spasticity

Post-traumatic stress disorder (PTSD)

Seizure disorder, including epilepsy

Medical Marijuana Law in New Mexico

New Mexico removed state-level criminal penalties for the use and possession of marijuana by qualifying patients with debilitating conditions in 2007.

It is legal for adults in New Mexico to use and possess up to two ounces of cannabis flower or 16 grams of concentrates in public and an unspecified amount at home.

PATIENT POSSESSION LIMITS:

Eight ounces (over a 90-day period)

HOME CULTIVATION:

Yes. 16 plants (no more than four mature at once)

STATE-LICENSED DISPENSARIES:

Yes

CAREGIVERS:

Yes. A primary caregiver is a person responsible for the well-being of a qualifying patient with respect to their use of marijuana. Primary caregivers must be residents of New Mexico and must be at least 18 years of age.

RECIPROCITY:

No

QUALIFYING CONDITIONS:

Alzheimer's disease

Amyotrophic Lateral Sclerosis (Lou Gehrig's disease)

Anorexia/cachexia

Autism spectrum disorder

Cancer

Cervical dystonia

Crohn's disease

Epilepsy and other seizure disorders

Friedreich's ataxia

Glaucoma

Hepatitis C infection

HIV/AIDS

Hospice patients

Huntington's disease

Inflammatory autoimmune-mediated arthritis

Intractable nausea/vomiting

Lewy body disease

Multiple sclerosis

Obstructive sleep apnea

Opioid dependency or other substance abuse disorders

Painful peripheral neuropathy

Parkinson's disease

Post-traumatic stress disorder

Severe chronic pain

Spasmodic torticollis

Spinal cord damage

Spinal muscular atrophy

Ulcerative colitis

Medical Marijuana Laws in New York

Medical marijuana in New York was signed into law in 2014. The law will automatically expire after seven years unless renewed by state legislature.

Marijuana is legalized for anyone 21 and older in New York. The general public can possess up to three ounces of cannabis and 24 grams of concentrates while registered patients are allowed a 60-day supply at any time.

HOME CULTIVATION:

No

STATE-LICENSED DISPENSARIES:

Yes. Initially, 5 producers of cannabis preparations and up to 20 dispensaries are permitted to be licensed by the state. In 2017, an additional 5 entities where licensed to cultivate and dispense marijuana.

PATIENT POSSESSION LIMITS:

60-day supply. Only non-smokable preparations are allowed

CAREGIVERS:

Yes. Each qualifying patients may have support of up to two caregivers, and each caregiver may not serve any more than five patients.

RECIPROCITY:

No

QUALIFYING CONDITIONS:

Acute pain management

Amyotrophic Lateral Sclerosis (ALS)

Cancer

Chronic pain

Epilepsy

HIV/AIDS

Huntington's Disease

Inflammatory bowel disease

Parkinson's Disease

Post-Traumatic Stress Disorder

Multiple Sclerosis

Neuropathies

Opioid substitution

Spinal cord damage

Medical Marijuana Law in North Carolina

Medical and recreational marijuana use is illegal in North Carolina. The state allows patients with intractable epilepsy to possess and consume CBD oil that contains less than 0.9% THC, though no regulated retail locations are operational.

North Carolina's CBD-only legislation calls for a trial study to be conducted by four universities in the state: UNC, Duke, Wake Forest and East Carolina.

The primary focus is to make CBD oil available to minors that suffer from seizures.

QUALIFYING CONDITIONS:

Intractable epilepsy

PATIENT POSSESSION LIMITS:

Cannabis extract containing less than nine-tenths of a percent THC and at least five percent CBD

HOME CULTIVATION:

No

STATE-LICENSED DISPENSARIES:

No

CAREGIVERS:

No

RECIPROCITY:

No

Medical Marijuana Law in North Dakota

It's illegal for adults to consume cannabis in North Dakota, but qualified patients are protected under the Compassionate Care Act. Those with a valid medical marijuana ID card can possess up to three grams of flower in a 30-day period. North Dakota recently reduced marijuana penalties for all, reclassifying possession of up to 14 grams of cannabis to a criminal infraction with no jail time.

PATIENT POSSESSION LIMITS:

Qualifying patients can legally possess three ounces of herbal cannabis.

HOME CULTIVATION:

No

STATE-LICENSED DISPENSARIES:

Yes. No more than two cultivators and eight dispensaries (not yet operational).

QUALIFYING CONDITIONS:

Agitation from Alzheimer's disease or related dementia

Amyotrophic lateral sclerosis (ALS)

Anorexia nervosa

Anxiety disorder

Autism spectrum disorder

Brain injury

Bulimia nervosa

Cachexia or Wasting syndrome

Cancer

Chronic or debilitating disease

Crohn's disease

Ehlers-Danlos syndrome

Endometriosis

Epilepsy

Fibromyalgia

Glaucoma

Hepatitis C

HIV/AIDS

Interstitial cystitis

Intractable nausea

Neuropathy

Migraine

Multiple sclerosis

Post-traumatic stress disorder (PTSD)

Rheumatoid arthritis

Seizures

Severe and persistent muscle spasms

Severe debilitating pain

Spinal stenosis

Tourette syndrome

Medical Marijuana Law in Ohio

Only registered patients can legally consume and possess marijuana in Ohio. Possession is limited to a 45-day supply from a licensed dispensary, though possession of less than 3.5 ounces is considered a minor misdemeanor for all.

HOME CULTIVATION:

No

STATE-LICENSED DISPENSARIES:

Yes, but they are not yet operational.

CAREGIVERS:

No

RECIPROCITY:

Not specified

QUALIFYING CONDITIONS:

Acquired immune deficiency syndrome (AIDS)

Alzheimer's disease

Amyotrophic lateral sclerosis (Lou Gehrig's disease)

Arthritis*

Cachexia

Cancer

Chronic migraines*

Chronic traumatic encephalopathy

Complex regional pain syndrome*

Crohn's disease

Epilepsy or other seizure disorders

Fibromyalgia

Glaucoma

Hepatitis C

Inflammatory bowel disease

Multiple Sclerosis

Pain that is either of the following nature: (i) Chronic and severe; or (ii) Intractable

Parkinson's disease

Positive status for HIV

Post-traumatic stress disorder

Sickle cell anemia

Spinal cord disease or injury

Tourette's syndrome

Traumatic brain injury

Ulcerative colitis

PATIENT POSSESSION LIMITS:

Not yet specified. Cannabis products can be dispensed as oils, tinctures, edibles, patches or herbal matter.

Medical Marijuana Law in Oklahoma

Oklahoma introduced legislation allowing CBD oil in 2015 for epileptic children. A more comprehensive medical marijuana law, allowing full-plant marijuana use for a range of conditions, was introduced in 2018.

Recreational marijuana is illegal in Oklahoma, but patients may use cannabis to treat a list of qualifying conditions. Those registered with the state can legally possess up to three ounces of cannabis in public and eight ounces at home, one ounce of cannabis concentrates, and 72 ounces of edible products. Patients are permitted to cultivate their own cannabis at home but cannot exceed six mature plants and six seedlings.

QUALIFYING CONDITIONS:

Any condition as recommended by the treating physician.

PATIENT POSSESSION LIMITS:

Eight ounces of marijuana in their residence, one ounce of concentrated marijuana, 72 ounces of edible marijuana, and up to three ounces of marijuana on the person.

HOME CULTIVATION:

Yes. Six mature plants and six immature seedlings are permitted.

STATE-LICENSED DISPENSARIES:

Yes

CAREGIVERS:

Yes. Qualified caregivers may provide support for a homebound licensed patient.

RECIPROCITY:

No

Medical Marijuana Law in Oregon

Marijuana is legal in Oregon. Possession
  limits for recreational users are one ounce of
  flower and five grams of concentrates, while
  patients and caregivers are permitted 24
  ounces of flower and 5 grams of extracts.
  Both can legally grow marijuana at home
  under certain restriction.

Oregon medical marijuana laws allow use,
  possession and cultivation by qualifying
  patients. Patients must possess a signed
  recommendation from a physician
  confirming marijuana "may mitigate" his or
  her debilitating disease.

HOME CULTIVATION:

Yes. Six mature plants are allowed, as well
  as up to 18 immature seedlings.

STATE-LICENSED DISPENSARIES:

Yes. A directory of state-licensed
  dispensaries can be found at oregon.gov

CAREGIVERS:

Yes. A primary caregiver is a person who is
  responsible for managing the well-being of a
  qualifying patient diagnosed with a
  debilitating medical condition. A primary

caregiver must be at least 18 years of age and must not be the patient's physician. A patient can only have one primary caregiver at any one time.

QUALIFYING CONDITIONS:

Alzheimer's disease

Cachexia

Cancer

Chronic pain

Glaucoma

HIV or AIDS

Nausea

Persistent muscle spasms

Post-traumatic stress

Seizures

Other conditions are subject to approval

PATIENT POSSESSION LIMITS:

Twenty-four ounces of usable marijuana

RECIPROCITY:

No

Medical Marijuana Law in Rhode Island

Rhode Island's medical marijuana law became effective in 2006, allowing the medicinal use, possession and cultivation of cannabis for qualifying patients.

Only patients registered with the state's medical marijuana program can legally use and possess up to 2.5 ounces of cannabis. The program allows home cultivation with a limit of 12 mature plants and 12 seedlings. Recreational possession of one ounce or less is considered a civil crime for first-time offenders.

PATIENT POSSESSION LIMITS:

Two and a half ounces

HOME CULTIVATION:

Yes. Up to 12 mature plants and 12 seedlings are permitted within an indoor facility.

Two or more cardholders are permitted to cooperate in the cultivation of cannabis in residential/non-residential locations subject to the following:

Non-residential – no more than 10 ounces of useable cannabis, 48 mature plants and 48 seedlings are allowed.

Residential – no more than 10 ounces of usable cannabis, 24 mature plants and 24 seedlings are allowed.

STATE-LICENSED DISPENSARIES:

Yes, no more than nine are allowed

CAREGIVERS:

Yes. Caregivers must be aged 21 or older and a primary caregiver may assist no more than five qualifying patients at any one time.

RECIPROCITY:

Yes. Patients with a debilitating medical condition and a registry identification card are permitted to engage in the medical use of cannabis.

cultivation of cannabis for qualifying patients.

QUALIFYING CONDITIONS:

Alzheimer's Disease

Autism

Cachexia

Cancer

Chronic pain

Crohn's disease

Glaucoma

Hepatitis C

HIV/AIDS

Nausea

Persistent muscle spasms

Post-traumatic stress disorder

Seizures

Other conditions are subject to approval

Medical Marijuana Law in South Carolina

CBD legislation was passed in South Carolina in 2014. The bill requires the University of South Carolina to establish a clinical trial to research the effectiveness of CBD oil in treating debilitating conditions. All forms of marijuana are illegal in South Carolina. In 2014 the state approved use of prescribed CBD products containing less than 0.9% THC by patients suffering from a limited list of conditions.

PATIENT POSSESSION LIMITS:

Cannabis extracts are permitted if they contain less than nine-tenths of a percent THC and more than 15 percent CBD

HOME CULTIVATION:

No

STATE-LICENSED DISPENSARIES:

No

CAREGIVERS:

No

RECIPROCITY:

No

QUALIFYING CONDITIONS:

Dravet Syndrome

Lennox-Gastaut Syndrome

Refractory epilepsy

Medical Marijuana Law in South Dakota

As of July 2021, cannabis is legal for both recreational and medical use. Adults may possess up to one ounce of cannabis with no more than eight grams in concentrated form. However, there are currently no operational dispensaries in South Dakota.

PATIENT POSSESSION LIMITS

Medical marijuana patients may possess up to three ounces of cannabis including other allowable products. Specifics to be determined within 120 days on the bill coming into effect.

HOME CULTIVATION

Yes, up to three plants. In certain circumstances, a physician may authorize a patient to cultivate greater quantities.

CAREGIVERS

Yes. All caregivers must submit the proper required documentation to the State Department of Health.

QUALIFYING CONDITIONS

AIDS/HIV

Amyotrophic lateral sclerosis (ALS)

Multiple sclerosis

Cancer associated with severe or chronic
pain, nausea or severe vomiting, or
cachexia or severe wasting

Crohn's disease

Epilepsy and seizures

Glaucoma

Post-Traumatic Stress Disorder (PTSD)

Other medical condition or its treatment
may be added by the Department of Health.

Medical Marijuana Law in Tennessee

Adult-use is illegal, but the state does permit medical marijuana restricted to CBD products containing less than 0.9% THC. Possession of a half-ounce or less is considered a misdemeanor punishable by up to one year in jail.

PATIENT POSSESSION LIMITS:

Cannabis oil containing no more than nine-tenths of a percent THC.

HOME CULTIVATION:

No

STATE-LICENSED DISPENSARIES:

No

CAREGIVERS:

No

RECIPROCITY:

No

QUALIFYING CONDITIONS:

Intractable seizures

Alzheimer's disease

ALS

Cancer

Recalcitrant nausea and vomiting

Inflammatory bowel disease

Crohn's disease

Ulcerative colitis

Epilepsy or seizure

Multiple sclerosis

Parkinson's disease

Human immunodeficiency virus (HIV)

Acquired immunodeficiency syndrome (AIDS)

Sickle cell disease

Medical Marijuana Law in Texas

Texas is home to a limited medical marijuana program that allows patients use of low-THC cannabis containing not more than .5% THC. Smoking is prohibited under the medical marijuana law and all patients must register with the state. Texas allows medical marijuana in its most limited form; non-intoxicating CBD oil Possession of even small amounts of marijuana may result in severe criminal penalties.

PATIENT POSSESSION LIMITS:

Cannabis extracts that are high in CBD and have less than 0.5 percent THC.

HOME CULTIVATION:

No

STATE-LICENSED DISPENSARIES:

Yes, up to three licensed dispensaries.

CAREGIVERS:

No

RECIPROCITY:

No

QUALIFYING CONDITIONS:

Autism

Amyotrophic lateral sclerosis

Incurable neurodegenerative disorders

Intractable Epilepsy

Multiple sclerosis

Seizure disorders

Terminal cancer

Medical Marijuana Law in Utah

Recreational marijuana is not legal or decriminalized in Utah. In 2018 voters passed a medical marijuana law that allows patients to use medical marijuana purchased from licensed dispensaries. Patients may possess up to 112 grams of cannabis within a 30-day period. Non-patients in possession of small amounts could face up to six months imprisonment and a $1,000 fine.

PATIENT POSSESSION LIMITS:

Medical cannabis products can come in the following forms: tablets, capsules, concentrated oils, topical preparations, transdermal preparations, sublingual preparations, liquid suspensions, or gelatinous cubes or lozenges. There is a state-mandated "legal dosage limit" of 20 grams of THC per single dose. Cannabis flower must be dispensed in a "tamper-resistant" sealed container with a 60-day expiration date. Patients are permitted to obtain up to a 30-day supply of medical marijuana products. A 30-day supply of "unprocessed cannabis" should not exceed 113 grams by weight.

HOME CULTIVATION:

No. Replacement legislation enacted by the House and Senate rewrote the Utah Medical Cannabis Act to prohibit home grows.

STATE-LICENSED DISPENSARIES:

Yes, although they are defined as 'medical pharmacies' under the replacement legislation. No more than seven medical pharmacy licenses may be issued.

CAREGIVERS:

Yes. A patient may designate a maximum of two caregivers, who are permitted to purchase, transport, or otherwise assist the patient with his/her use of medicine.

QUALIFYING CONDITIONS:

ALS (Lou Gehrig's disease)

Alzheimer's disease

Autism

Cachexia

Cancer

Crohn's disease or ulcerative colitis

HIV/AIDS

Epilepsy or a similar condition that causes "debilitating seizures"

Multiple sclerosis or persistent and debilitating muscle spasms

Nausea (must be persistent)

Pain lasting longer than two weeks that is not adequately managed despite treatment attempts

PTSD "that is being treated or monitored by a licensed mental health therapist"

Any terminal illness where life expectancy is less than six months

Any condition resulting in hospice care

Any rare condition that effects fewer than 200,000 persons in the United States as defined by Section 526 of the Federal Food, Drug and Cosmetic Act and is not adequately managed despite treatment attempts

**Patients with a qualifying illness between the ages of 18 and 21 must petition the Compassionate Use Board for medical cannabis approval.

Medical Marijuana Law in Vermont

Vermont's medical marijuana law removed state-level criminal penalties for the use, possession and cultivation of marijuana by qualifying patients. Both medical marijuana and adult-use is legal. Recreational retail establishments are set to open in 2022, with limitations on the percentage of THC in flower and concentrates. Adults can possess up to one ounce or 5 grams of hashish, and registered patients can possess up to two ounces. Both can cultivate at home within limits.

PATIENT POSSESSION LIMITS:

Two ounces of usable marijuana

HOME CULTIVATION:

Yes. No more than nine marijuana plants are permitted, and only two may be mature at any one time.

STATE-LICENSED DISPENSARIES:

Yes. No more than five, a limit which increases to six when the program includes more than 7000 patients. Dispensaries are legally allowed to engage in home delivery.

CAREGIVERS:

Yes. A caregiver is a person who is responsible for managing the well-being of a qualifying patient in regard to their medicinal use of marijuana. A registered caregiver must never have been convicted of a drug-related crime and must be at least 21 years of age. Patients may only have one registered caregiver at a time, and the caregiver can only serve one patient.

RECIPROCITY:

No

QUALIFYING CONDITIONS:

Any patient receiving hospice care

Cachexia or wasting syndrome

Cancer

Crohn's disease

Glaucoma

HIV or AIDS

Multiple Sclerosis

Parkinson's disease

PTSD

Seizures

Severe or chronic pain

Severe nausea

Medical Marijuana Law in Virginia

Marijuana is legal for recreational use in Virginia. Medical marijuana is legal in Virginia since the state passed a law in 2020. Adults are permitted to possess up to one ounce of marijuana and cultivate four plants per household, though retail sales won't be operational until 2024. Registered patients are limited to cannabis oil with at least 5 mg of CBD and no more than 10 mg THC. Possession is not to exceed a 90-day supply.

PATIENT POSSESSION LIMITS:

The specified possession limit of botanical cannabis is 4 ounces per 30 days. The specified possession limit for cannabis oil is a 90-day supply.

HOME CULTIVATION:

No

STATE-LICENSED DISPENSARIES:

Yes

CAREGIVERS:

Qualifying patients may have a "registered agent", an individual designated by a patient who has been issued a written certification, or, if such patient is a minor or an incapacitated adult, designated by such patient's parent or legal guardian, and registered with the Board pursuant to subsection G.

RECIPROCITY:

No

QUALIFYING CONDITIONS:

Any diagnosed condition or disease that a physician determines will benefit from the use of marijuana.

Medical Marijuana Law in Washington

Recreational marijuana laws that took effect in 2012 allow adults to possess up to one ounce of usable marijuana and seven grams of concentrates. Patients registered with the state's authorization database are permitted to purchase and possess up to three ounces of marijuana and 21 grams of concentrates.

Washington State's medical marijuana law, enacted by ballot initiative in 1998, removed state-level penalties for the use, possession and cultivation of marijuana by qualifying patients.

"Qualifying patients" refers to those who have valid documentation from their physician stating that the "potential benefits of the medical use of marijuana would likely outweigh the health risks."

PATIENT POSSESSION LIMITS:

Those in the voluntary patient database are permitted to possess: 48 ounces of marijuana-infused product in solid form, 3 ounces of useable marijuana, 216 ounces of marijuana-infused product in liquid form, or 21 grams of marijuana concentrates.

HOME CULTIVATION:

Those in the voluntary patient database may cultivate up to six plants for personal medical use and may possess up to 8 ounces of usable marijuana produced from the plants. If a physician confirms that the medical needs of the patient exceed these limits, he or she will be able to grow up to 15 plants, yielding up to 16 ounces of usable marijuana, for the medicinal use of the patient.

If a patient has not been entered into the medical marijuana database, he or she may grow up to four plants for personal medicinal use and may possess up to six ounces of usable marijuana.

STATE-LICENSED DISPENSARIES:

No. Retail providers may engage in the sale of medical marijuana.

CAREGIVERS:

Yes. A designated caregiver is a person who has been confirmed in writing by a patient to serve as their primary caregiver. Caregivers must be at least 21 years or age. Providers must either possess authorization from the patient's physician or must be entered into an authorized database. The provider is only allowed to provide cannabis to the specified patient.

RECIPROCITY:

No

QUALIFYING CONDITIONS:

Cachexia

Cancer

Crohn's disease

Glaucoma

Hepatitis C

HIV or AIDS

Intractable pain

Persistent muscle spasms, and/or spasticity

Nausea

Post-Traumatic Stress Disorder

Seizures

Traumatic Brain Injury

Any "terminal or debilitating condition"

Medical Marijuana Law in West Virginia

Recreational laws in West Virginia are strict, and a first-time possession charge is punishable by a minimum of 90 days incarceration. Medical marijuana patients who are registered with the Bureau of Health may purchase marijuana from a licensed dispensary and possess up to a 30-day supply which is determined per patient. A comprehensive medical marijuana law has been signed in by Gov. Jim Justice, although the new program is not yet operational. The Bureau of Public Health will begin to issue marijuana patient ID cards on July 1, 2019.

PATIENT POSSESSION LIMITS:

Patients are allowed to possess a "30-day supply" of cannabis-infused products. Patients can obtain medical marijuana in any of the following forms:

Flower

Oils

Tinctures

Pills

Topicals

Patches

HOME CULTIVATION:

No

STATE-LICENSED DISPENSARIES:

Yes

CAREGIVERS:

Yes. A qualified medical marijuana patient may designate no more than two caregivers. Each caregiver can serve a maximum of five patients at any one time.

RECIPROCITY:

Yes, only for terminally ill patients.

QUALIFYING CONDITIONS:

Amyotrophic lateral sclerosis

Cancer

Crohn's disease

HIV/AIDS

Epilepsy

Huntington's disease

Intractable seizures

Multiple sclerosis

Neuropathies (chronic nerve pain)

Parkinson's disease

Post-traumatic stress disorder

Severe chronic or intractable pain

Spinal cord damage

Sickle cell anemia.

Terminal illness

Marijuana Law in Wisconsin

Restricted medical marijuana use is legal in Wisconsin. The law allows patients with a doctor's certification to treat unspecified conditions with CBD oil. Possession of cannabis for any use is illegal. Wisconsin legalized the medicinal use of CBD oil for the treatment of seizures in 2014, but it still remains difficult for patients to access it.

QUALIFYING CONDITIONS:

Any medical condition which a physician recommends it for

PATIENT POSSESSION LIMITS:

Possession of any form of cannabidiol without a psychoactive effect

HOME CULTIVATION:

No

Medical STATE-LICENSED DISPENSARIES:

No

CAREGIVERS:

No

RECIPROCITY:

No

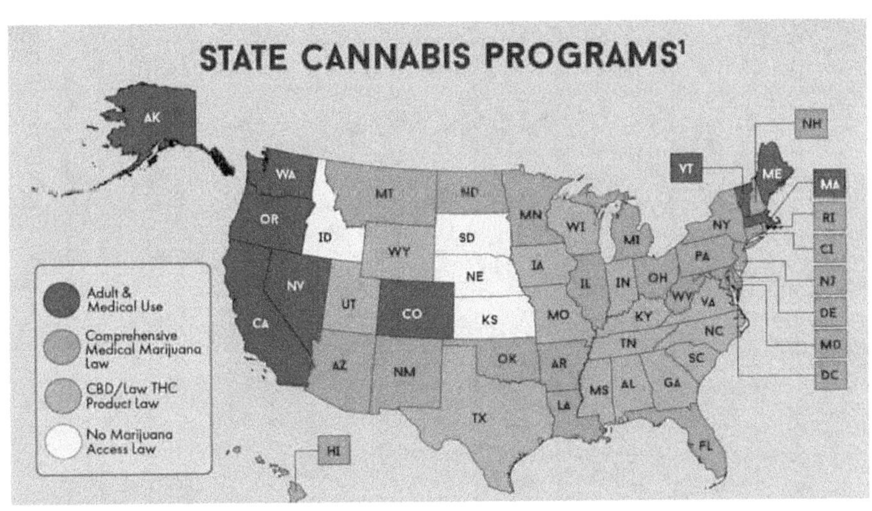

STATE CANNABIS PROGRAMS[1]
AK
WA
OR
ID
NV
CA
UT
AZ
NM
MT
WY
CO
MT
ND
SD
NE
KS
OK
TX
MN
IA
MO
AR
LA
WI
IL
MS
IN
KY
TN
AL
MI
OH
WV
GA
VA
NC
SC
FL
NY
PA
NH
VT
ME
MA
RI
CT
NJ
DE
MD
DC
HI
Adult & Medical Use
Comprehensive Medical Marijuana Law
CBD/Law THC Product Law
No Marijuana Access Law

www.ingramcontent.com/pod-product-compliance
Lightning Source LLC
Chambersburg PA
CBHW050531160726
48003CB00002B/543